FOOD JOURNAL

Breakfast

	Servings	Calories
	Subtotal	

Snack

	Subtotal	

Lunch

	Subtotal	

Snack

	Subtotal	

Dinner

	Subtotal	

Snack

	Subtotal	

Total Calories From Food [   ]

FITNESS ACTIVITY JOURNAL

	Duration	Calories

Total Calories From Fitness [   ]

NOTES

FOOD JOURNAL

Breakfast	Servings	Calories
	Subtotal	

Snack		
	Subtotal	

Lunch		
	Subtotal	

Snack		
	Subtotal	

Dinner		
	Subtotal	

Snack		
	Subtotal	

	Total Calories From Food	

FITNESS ACTIVITY JOURNAL

	Duration	Calories
Total Calories From Fitness		

NOTES

FOOD JOURNAL

Breakfast	Servings	Calories
	Subtotal	
Snack		
	Subtotal	
Lunch		
	Subtotal	
Snack		
	Subtotal	
Dinner		
	Subtotal	
Snack		
	Subtotal	
	Total Calories From Food	

FITNESS ACTIVITY JOURNAL

	Duration	Calories
	Total Calories From Fitness	

NOTES

FOOD JOURNAL

Breakfast	Servings	Calories
	Subtotal	

Snack		
	Subtotal	

Lunch		
	Subtotal	

Snack		
	Subtotal	

Dinner		
	Subtotal	

Snack		
	Subtotal	

Total Calories From Food

FITNESS ACTIVITY JOURNAL

	Duration	Calories

Total Calories From Fitness

NOTES

FOOD JOURNAL

Breakfast	Servings	Calories
	Subtotal	

Snack		
	Subtotal	

Lunch		
	Subtotal	

Snack		
	Subtotal	

Dinner		
	Subtotal	

Snack		
	Subtotal	

Total Calories From Food

FITNESS ACTIVITY JOURNAL

	Duration	Calories

Total Calories From Fitness

NOTES

FOOD JOURNAL

Breakfast	Servings	Calories
	Subtotal	

Snack		
	Subtotal	

Lunch		
	Subtotal	

Snack		
	Subtotal	

Dinner		
	Subtotal	

Snack		
	Subtotal	

Total Calories From Food

FITNESS ACTIVITY JOURNAL

	Duration	Calories

Total Calories From Fitness

NOTES

FOOD JOURNAL

Breakfast	Servings	Calories
	Subtotal	

Snack		
	Subtotal	

Lunch		
	Subtotal	

Snack		
	Subtotal	

Dinner		
	Subtotal	

Snack		
	Subtotal	

Total Calories From Food [   ]

FITNESS ACTIVITY JOURNAL

	Duration	Calories

Total Calories From Fitness [   ]

NOTES

_____

_____

_____

_____

_____

FOOD JOURNAL

Breakfast	Servings	Calories
	Subtotal	

Snack		
	Subtotal	

Lunch		
	Subtotal	

Snack		
	Subtotal	

Dinner		
	Subtotal	

Snack		
	Subtotal	
	Total Calories From Food	

FITNESS ACTIVITY JOURNAL

	Duration	Calories
	Total Calories From Fitness	

NOTES

FOOD JOURNAL

Breakfast	Servings	Calories
	Subtotal	

Snack		
	Subtotal	

Lunch		
	Subtotal	

Snack		
	Subtotal	

Dinner		
	Subtotal	

Snack		
	Subtotal	

Total Calories From Food [   ]

FITNESS ACTIVITY JOURNAL

	Duration	Calories

Total Calories From Fitness [   ]

NOTES

FOOD JOURNAL

Breakfast	Servings	Calories
	Subtotal	

Snack		
	Subtotal	

Lunch		
	Subtotal	

Snack		
	Subtotal	

Dinner		
	Subtotal	

Snack		
	Subtotal	

Total Calories From Food [   ]

FITNESS ACTIVITY JOURNAL

	Duration	Calories

Total Calories From Fitness [   ]

NOTES

FOOD JOURNAL

Breakfast	Servings	Calories
	Subtotal	

Snack		
	Subtotal	

Lunch		
	Subtotal	

Snack		
	Subtotal	

Dinner		
	Subtotal	

Snack		
	Subtotal	

Total Calories From Food

FITNESS ACTIVITY JOURNAL

	Duration	Calories

Total Calories From Fitness

NOTES

FOOD JOURNAL

Breakfast	Servings	Calories
	Subtotal	
Snack		
	Subtotal	
Lunch		
	Subtotal	
Snack		
	Subtotal	
Dinner		
	Subtotal	
Snack		
	Subtotal	

Total Calories From Food

FITNESS ACTIVITY JOURNAL

	Duration	Calories

Total Calories From Fitness

NOTES

FOOD JOURNAL

Breakfast	Servings	Calories
	Subtotal	

Snack		
	Subtotal	

Lunch		
	Subtotal	

Snack		
	Subtotal	

Dinner		
	Subtotal	

Snack		
	Subtotal	

Total Calories From Food [   ]

FITNESS ACTIVITY JOURNAL

	Duration	Calories

Total Calories From Fitness [   ]

NOTES

FOOD JOURNAL

Breakfast	Servings	Calories
	Subtotal	

Snack		
	Subtotal	

Lunch		
	Subtotal	

Snack		
	Subtotal	

Dinner		
	Subtotal	

Snack		
	Subtotal	

Total Calories From Food

FITNESS ACTIVITY JOURNAL

	Duration	Calories

Total Calories From Fitness

NOTES

FOOD JOURNAL

Breakfast	Servings	Calories
	Subtotal	

Snack		
	Subtotal	

Lunch		
	Subtotal	

Snack		
	Subtotal	

Dinner		
	Subtotal	

Snack		
	Subtotal	

Total Calories From Food

FITNESS ACTIVITY JOURNAL

	Duration	Calories

Total Calories From Fitness

NOTES

FOOD JOURNAL

Breakfast	Servings	Calories
	Subtotal	

Snack		
	Subtotal	

Lunch		
	Subtotal	

Snack		
	Subtotal	

Dinner		
	Subtotal	

Snack		
	Subtotal	

Total Calories From Food

FITNESS ACTIVITY JOURNAL

	Duration	Calories

Total Calories From Fitness

NOTES

FOOD JOURNAL

Breakfast	Servings	Calories
	Subtotal	
Snack		
	Subtotal	
Lunch		
	Subtotal	
Snack		
	Subtotal	
Dinner		
	Subtotal	
Snack		
	Subtotal	

Total Calories From Food ☐

FITNESS ACTIVITY JOURNAL

	Duration	Calories

Total Calories From Fitness ☐

NOTES

FOOD JOURNAL

Breakfast	Servings	Calories
	Subtotal	

Snack		
	Subtotal	

Lunch		
	Subtotal	

Snack		
	Subtotal	

Dinner		
	Subtotal	

Snack		
	Subtotal	

Total Calories From Food

FITNESS ACTIVITY JOURNAL

	Duration	Calories

Total Calories From Fitness

NOTES

FOOD JOURNAL

Breakfast	Servings	Calories
	Subtotal	

Snack		
	Subtotal	

Lunch		
	Subtotal	

Snack		
	Subtotal	

Dinner		
	Subtotal	

Snack		
	Subtotal	

Total Calories From Food

FITNESS ACTIVITY JOURNAL

	Duration	Calories

Total Calories From Fitness

NOTES

FOOD JOURNAL

Breakfast	Servings	Calories
	Subtotal	

Snack		
	Subtotal	

Lunch		
	Subtotal	

Snack		
	Subtotal	

Dinner		
	Subtotal	

Snack		
	Subtotal	

Total Calories From Food [＿＿＿＿＿＿]

FITNESS ACTIVITY JOURNAL

	Duration	Calories

Total Calories From Fitness [＿＿＿＿＿＿]

NOTES

FOOD JOURNAL

Breakfast	Servings	Calories
	Subtotal	

Snack		
	Subtotal	

Lunch		
	Subtotal	

Snack		
	Subtotal	

Dinner		
	Subtotal	

Snack		
	Subtotal	

Total Calories From Food

FITNESS ACTIVITY JOURNAL

	Duration	Calories

Total Calories From Fitness

NOTES

FOOD JOURNAL

Breakfast	Servings	Calories
	Subtotal	

Snack		
	Subtotal	

Lunch		
	Subtotal	

Snack		
	Subtotal	

Dinner		
	Subtotal	

Snack		
	Subtotal	

Total Calories From Food [_____]

FITNESS ACTIVITY JOURNAL

	Duration	Calories

Total Calories From Fitness [_____]

NOTES

FOOD JOURNAL

Breakfast	Servings	Calories
	Subtotal	

Snack		
	Subtotal	

Lunch		
	Subtotal	

Snack		
	Subtotal	

Dinner		
	Subtotal	

Snack		
	Subtotal	

Total Calories From Food

FITNESS ACTIVITY JOURNAL

	Duration	Calories

Total Calories From Fitness

NOTES

FOOD JOURNAL

Breakfast	Servings	Calories
	Subtotal	

Snack		
	Subtotal	

Lunch		
	Subtotal	

Snack		
	Subtotal	

Dinner		
	Subtotal	

Snack		
	Subtotal	

Total Calories From Food

FITNESS ACTIVITY JOURNAL

	Duration	Calories

Total Calories From Fitness

NOTES

FOOD JOURNAL

Breakfast	Servings	Calories
	Subtotal	

Snack		
	Subtotal	

Lunch		
	Subtotal	

Snack		
	Subtotal	

Dinner		
	Subtotal	

Snack		
	Subtotal	

Total Calories From Food [   ]

FITNESS ACTIVITY JOURNAL

	Duration	Calories

Total Calories From Fitness [   ]

NOTES

FOOD JOURNAL

Breakfast	Servings	Calories
	Subtotal	

Snack		
	Subtotal	

Lunch		
	Subtotal	

Snack		
	Subtotal	

Dinner		
	Subtotal	

Snack		
	Subtotal	

Total Calories From Food

FITNESS ACTIVITY JOURNAL

	Duration	Calories

Total Calories From Fitness

NOTES

FOOD JOURNAL

Breakfast	Servings	Calories
	Subtotal	

Snack		
	Subtotal	

Lunch		
	Subtotal	

Snack		
	Subtotal	

Dinner		
	Subtotal	

Snack		
	Subtotal	

Total Calories From Food

FITNESS ACTIVITY JOURNAL

	Duration	Calories

Total Calories From Fitness

NOTES

FOOD JOURNAL

Breakfast	Servings	Calories
	Subtotal	

Snack		
	Subtotal	

Lunch		
	Subtotal	

Snack		
	Subtotal	

Dinner		
	Subtotal	

Snack		
	Subtotal	

Total Calories From Food

FITNESS ACTIVITY JOURNAL

	Duration	Calories

Total Calories From Fitness

NOTES

FOOD JOURNAL

Breakfast	Servings	Calories
	Subtotal	

Snack		
	Subtotal	

Lunch		
	Subtotal	

Snack		
	Subtotal	

Dinner		
	Subtotal	

Snack		
	Subtotal	

Total Calories From Food

FITNESS ACTIVITY JOURNAL

	Duration	Calories

Total Calories From Fitness

NOTES

FOOD JOURNAL

Breakfast	Servings	Calories
	Subtotal	

Snack		
	Subtotal	

Lunch		
	Subtotal	

Snack		
	Subtotal	

Dinner		
	Subtotal	

Snack		
	Subtotal	

Total Calories From Food

FITNESS ACTIVITY JOURNAL

	Duration	Calories

Total Calories From Fitness

NOTES

FOOD JOURNAL

Breakfast	Servings	Calories
	Subtotal	

Snack		
	Subtotal	

Lunch		
	Subtotal	

Snack		
	Subtotal	

Dinner		
	Subtotal	

Snack		
	Subtotal	

	Total Calories From Food	

FITNESS ACTIVITY JOURNAL

	Duration	Calories
	Total Calories From Fitness	

NOTES

FOOD JOURNAL

Breakfast	Servings	Calories
	Subtotal	

Snack		
	Subtotal	

Lunch		
	Subtotal	

Snack		
	Subtotal	

Dinner		
	Subtotal	

Snack		
	Subtotal	

Total Calories From Food [_____]

FITNESS ACTIVITY JOURNAL

	Duration	Calories

Total Calories From Fitness [_____]

NOTES

FOOD JOURNAL

Breakfast	Servings	Calories
	Subtotal	

Snack		
	Subtotal	

Lunch		
	Subtotal	

Snack		
	Subtotal	

Dinner		
	Subtotal	

Snack		
	Subtotal	

Total Calories From Food

FITNESS ACTIVITY JOURNAL

	Duration	Calories

Total Calories From Fitness

NOTES

FOOD JOURNAL

Breakfast	Servings	Calories
	Subtotal	

Snack		
	Subtotal	

Lunch		
	Subtotal	

Snack		
	Subtotal	

Dinner		
	Subtotal	

Snack		
	Subtotal	

Total Calories From Food

FITNESS ACTIVITY JOURNAL

	Duration	Calories

Total Calories From Fitness

NOTES

FOOD JOURNAL

Breakfast	Servings	Calories
	Subtotal	

Snack		
	Subtotal	

Lunch		
	Subtotal	

Snack		
	Subtotal	

Dinner		
	Subtotal	

Snack		
	Subtotal	

Total Calories From Food [ ]

FITNESS ACTIVITY JOURNAL

	Duration	Calories

Total Calories From Fitness [ ]

NOTES

FOOD JOURNAL

Breakfast	Servings	Calories
	Subtotal	

Snack		
	Subtotal	

Lunch		
	Subtotal	

Snack		
	Subtotal	

Dinner		
	Subtotal	

Snack		
	Subtotal	

Total Calories From Food

FITNESS ACTIVITY JOURNAL

	Duration	Calories

Total Calories From Fitness

NOTES

FOOD JOURNAL

Breakfast		Servings	Calories
		Subtotal	

Snack			
		Subtotal	

Lunch			
		Subtotal	

Snack			
		Subtotal	

Dinner			
		Subtotal	

Snack			
		Subtotal	

Total Calories From Food [   ]

FITNESS ACTIVITY JOURNAL

	Duration	Calories

Total Calories From Fitness [   ]

NOTES

FOOD JOURNAL

Breakfast	Servings	Calories
	Subtotal	

Snack		
	Subtotal	

Lunch		
	Subtotal	

Snack		
	Subtotal	

Dinner		
	Subtotal	

Snack		
	Subtotal	

Total Calories From Food

FITNESS ACTIVITY JOURNAL

	Duration	Calories

Total Calories From Fitness

NOTES

FOOD JOURNAL

Breakfast	Servings	Calories
	Subtotal	

Snack		
	Subtotal	

Lunch		
	Subtotal	

Snack		
	Subtotal	

Dinner		
	Subtotal	

Snack		
	Subtotal	

	Total Calories From Food	

FITNESS ACTIVITY JOURNAL

	Duration	Calories
	Total Calories From Fitness	

NOTES

_____

_____

_____

_____

_____

_____

FOOD JOURNAL

Breakfast	Servings	Calories
	Subtotal	

Snack		
	Subtotal	

Lunch		
	Subtotal	

Snack		
	Subtotal	

Dinner		
	Subtotal	

Snack		
	Subtotal	

Total Calories From Food

FITNESS ACTIVITY JOURNAL

	Duration	Calories

Total Calories From Fitness

NOTES

FOOD JOURNAL

Breakfast	Servings	Calories
	Subtotal	

Snack		
	Subtotal	

Lunch		
	Subtotal	

Snack		
	Subtotal	

Dinner		
	Subtotal	

Snack		
	Subtotal	

Total Calories From Food [   ]

FITNESS ACTIVITY JOURNAL

	Duration	Calories

Total Calories From Fitness [   ]

NOTES

_____

_____

_____

_____

_____

_____

FOOD JOURNAL

Breakfast	Servings	Calories
	Subtotal	

Snack		
	Subtotal	

Lunch		
	Subtotal	

Snack		
	Subtotal	

Dinner		
	Subtotal	

Snack		
	Subtotal	

Total Calories From Food

FITNESS ACTIVITY JOURNAL

	Duration	Calories

Total Calories From Fitness

NOTES

FOOD JOURNAL

Breakfast		Servings	Calories
		Subtotal	
Snack			
		Subtotal	
Lunch			
		Subtotal	
Snack			
		Subtotal	
Dinner			
		Subtotal	
Snack			
		Subtotal	
	Total Calories From Food		

FITNESS ACTIVITY JOURNAL

	Duration	Calories
Total Calories From Fitness		

NOTES

FOOD JOURNAL

Breakfast	Servings	Calories
	Subtotal	

Snack	Servings	Calories
	Subtotal	

Lunch	Servings	Calories
	Subtotal	

Snack	Servings	Calories
	Subtotal	

Dinner	Servings	Calories
	Subtotal	

Snack	Servings	Calories
	Subtotal	

Total Calories From Food

FITNESS ACTIVITY JOURNAL

	Duration	Calories

Total Calories From Fitness

NOTES

FOOD JOURNAL

Breakfast	Servings	Calories
	Subtotal	

Snack		
	Subtotal	

Lunch		
	Subtotal	

Snack		
	Subtotal	

Dinner		
	Subtotal	

Snack		
	Subtotal	

Total Calories From Food

FITNESS ACTIVITY JOURNAL

	Duration	Calories

Total Calories From Fitness

NOTES

FOOD JOURNAL

Breakfast	Servings	Calories
	Subtotal	

Snack		
	Subtotal	

Lunch		
	Subtotal	

Snack		
	Subtotal	

Dinner		
	Subtotal	

Snack		
	Subtotal	

Total Calories From Food [ ]

FITNESS ACTIVITY JOURNAL

	Duration	Calories

Total Calories From Fitness [ ]

NOTES

FOOD JOURNAL

Breakfast	Servings	Calories
	Subtotal	

Snack		
	Subtotal	

Lunch		
	Subtotal	

Snack		
	Subtotal	

Dinner		
	Subtotal	

Snack		
	Subtotal	

Total Calories From Food

FITNESS ACTIVITY JOURNAL

	Duration	Calories

Total Calories From Fitness

NOTES

FOOD JOURNAL

Breakfast	Servings	Calories
	Subtotal	

Snack		
	Subtotal	

Lunch		
	Subtotal	

Snack		
	Subtotal	

Dinner		
	Subtotal	

Snack		
	Subtotal	

Total Calories From Food

FITNESS ACTIVITY JOURNAL

	Duration	Calories

Total Calories From Fitness

NOTES

FOOD JOURNAL

Breakfast	Servings	Calories
	Subtotal	

Snack		
	Subtotal	

Lunch		
	Subtotal	

Snack		
	Subtotal	

Dinner		
	Subtotal	

Snack		
	Subtotal	

Total Calories From Food

FITNESS ACTIVITY JOURNAL

	Duration	Calories

Total Calories From Fitness

NOTES

FOOD JOURNAL

Breakfast	Servings	Calories
	Subtotal	

Snack		
	Subtotal	

Lunch		
	Subtotal	

Snack		
	Subtotal	

Dinner		
	Subtotal	

Snack		
	Subtotal	

Total Calories From Food [   ]

FITNESS ACTIVITY JOURNAL

	Duration	Calories

Total Calories From Fitness [   ]

NOTES

FOOD JOURNAL

Breakfast	Servings	Calories	
		Subtotal	

Snack			
		Subtotal	

Lunch			
		Subtotal	

Snack			
		Subtotal	

Dinner			
		Subtotal	

Snack			
		Subtotal	

Total Calories From Food

FITNESS ACTIVITY JOURNAL

	Duration	Calories

Total Calories From Fitness

NOTES

_____

_____

_____

_____

_____

_____

_____

FOOD JOURNAL

Breakfast	Servings	Calories
	Subtotal	

Snack		
	Subtotal	

Lunch		
	Subtotal	

Snack		
	Subtotal	

Dinner		
	Subtotal	

Snack		
	Subtotal	

Total Calories From Food [   ]

FITNESS ACTIVITY JOURNAL

	Duration	Calories

Total Calories From Fitness [   ]

NOTES

FOOD JOURNAL

Breakfast	Servings	Calories
	Subtotal	

Snack		
	Subtotal	

Lunch		
	Subtotal	

Snack		
	Subtotal	

Dinner		
	Subtotal	

Snack		
	Subtotal	

Total Calories From Food

FITNESS ACTIVITY JOURNAL

	Duration	Calories

Total Calories From Fitness

NOTES

FOOD JOURNAL

Breakfast	Servings	Calories
	Subtotal	
Snack		
	Subtotal	
Lunch		
	Subtotal	
Snack		
	Subtotal	
Dinner		
	Subtotal	
Snack		
	Subtotal	
	Total Calories From Food	

FITNESS ACTIVITY JOURNAL

	Duration	Calories
	Total Calories From Fitness	

NOTES

FOOD JOURNAL

Breakfast	Servings	Calories
	Subtotal	

Snack		
	Subtotal	

Lunch		
	Subtotal	

Snack		
	Subtotal	

Dinner		
	Subtotal	

Snack		
	Subtotal	

Total Calories From Food	

FITNESS ACTIVITY JOURNAL

	Duration	Calories

Total Calories From Fitness	

NOTES

FOOD JOURNAL

Breakfast	Servings	Calories
	Subtotal	

Snack		
	Subtotal	

Lunch		
	Subtotal	

Snack		
	Subtotal	

Dinner		
	Subtotal	

Snack		
	Subtotal	

Total Calories From Food

FITNESS ACTIVITY JOURNAL

	Duration	Calories

Total Calories From Fitness

NOTES

FOOD JOURNAL

Breakfast	Servings	Calories
	Subtotal	

Snack		
	Subtotal	

Lunch		
	Subtotal	

Snack		
	Subtotal	

Dinner		
	Subtotal	

Snack		
	Subtotal	

	Total Calories From Food	

FITNESS ACTIVITY JOURNAL

	Duration	Calories
Total Calories From Fitness		

NOTES

FOOD JOURNAL

Breakfast	Servings	Calories
		Subtotal

Snack		
		Subtotal

Lunch		
		Subtotal

Snack		
		Subtotal

Dinner		
		Subtotal

Snack		
		Subtotal

Total Calories From Food

FITNESS ACTIVITY JOURNAL

	Duration	Calories

Total Calories From Fitness

NOTES

FOOD JOURNAL

Breakfast	Servings	Calories
	Subtotal	

Snack		
	Subtotal	

Lunch		
	Subtotal	

Snack		
	Subtotal	

Dinner		
	Subtotal	

Snack		
	Subtotal	

Total Calories From Food

FITNESS ACTIVITY JOURNAL

	Duration	Calories

Total Calories From Fitness

NOTES

FOOD JOURNAL

Breakfast	Servings	Calories
	Subtotal	
Snack		
	Subtotal	
Lunch		
	Subtotal	
Snack		
	Subtotal	
Dinner		
	Subtotal	
Snack		
	Subtotal	

Total Calories From Food [   ]

FITNESS ACTIVITY JOURNAL

	Duration	Calories

Total Calories From Fitness [   ]

NOTES

FOOD JOURNAL

Breakfast	Servings	Calories
	Subtotal	

Snack		
	Subtotal	

Lunch		
	Subtotal	

Snack		
	Subtotal	

Dinner		
	Subtotal	

Snack		
	Subtotal	

Total Calories From Food

FITNESS ACTIVITY JOURNAL

	Duration	Calories

Total Calories From Fitness

NOTES

FOOD JOURNAL

Breakfast   Servings Calories

Subtotal

Snack

Subtotal

Lunch

Subtotal

Snack

Subtotal

Dinner

Subtotal

Snack

Subtotal

Total Calories From Food

FITNESS ACTIVITY JOURNAL

Duration   Calories

Total Calories From Fitness

NOTES

FOOD JOURNAL

Breakfast	Servings	Calories
	Subtotal	

Snack		
	Subtotal	

Lunch		
	Subtotal	

Snack		
	Subtotal	

Dinner		
	Subtotal	

Snack		
	Subtotal	

Total Calories From Food

FITNESS ACTIVITY JOURNAL

	Duration	Calories

Total Calories From Fitness

NOTES

FOOD JOURNAL

Breakfast	Servings	Calories
	Subtotal	

Snack		
	Subtotal	

Lunch		
	Subtotal	

Snack		
	Subtotal	

Dinner		
	Subtotal	

Snack		
	Subtotal	

Total Calories From Food [   ]

FITNESS ACTIVITY JOURNAL

	Duration	Calories

Total Calories From Fitness [   ]

NOTES

FOOD JOURNAL

Breakfast	Servings	Calories
	Subtotal	

Snack		
	Subtotal	

Lunch		
	Subtotal	

Snack		
	Subtotal	

Dinner		
	Subtotal	

Snack		
	Subtotal	

Total Calories From Food

FITNESS ACTIVITY JOURNAL

	Duration	Calories

Total Calories From Fitness

NOTES

FOOD JOURNAL

Breakfast	Servings	Calories
	Subtotal	

Snack		
	Subtotal	

Lunch		
	Subtotal	

Snack		
	Subtotal	

Dinner		
	Subtotal	

Snack		
	Subtotal	

Total Calories From Food

FITNESS ACTIVITY JOURNAL

	Duration	Calories

Total Calories From Fitness

NOTES

FOOD JOURNAL

Breakfast	Servings	Calories
	Subtotal	

Snack		
	Subtotal	

Lunch		
	Subtotal	

Snack		
	Subtotal	

Dinner		
	Subtotal	

Snack		
	Subtotal	

Total Calories From Food

FITNESS ACTIVITY JOURNAL

	Duration	Calories

Total Calories From Fitness

NOTES

FOOD JOURNAL

Breakfast	Servings	Calories
	Subtotal	

Snack		
	Subtotal	

Lunch		
	Subtotal	

Snack		
	Subtotal	

Dinner		
	Subtotal	

Snack		
	Subtotal	

Total Calories From Food [   ]

FITNESS ACTIVITY JOURNAL

	Duration	Calories

Total Calories From Fitness [   ]

NOTES

FOOD JOURNAL

Breakfast	Servings	Calories
	Subtotal	

Snack		
	Subtotal	

Lunch		
	Subtotal	

Snack		
	Subtotal	

Dinner		
	Subtotal	

Snack		
	Subtotal	

Total Calories From Food

FITNESS ACTIVITY JOURNAL

	Duration	Calories

Total Calories From Fitness

NOTES

FOOD JOURNAL

Breakfast	Servings	Calories
	Subtotal	

Snack		
	Subtotal	

Lunch		
	Subtotal	

Snack		
	Subtotal	

Dinner		
	Subtotal	

Snack		
	Subtotal	

Total Calories From Food

FITNESS ACTIVITY JOURNAL

	Duration	Calories

Total Calories From Fitness

NOTES

FOOD JOURNAL

Breakfast	Servings	Calories
	Subtotal	

Snack		
	Subtotal	

Lunch		
	Subtotal	

Snack		
	Subtotal	

Dinner		
	Subtotal	

Snack		
	Subtotal	

Total Calories From Food

FITNESS ACTIVITY JOURNAL

	Duration	Calories

Total Calories From Fitness

NOTES

FOOD JOURNAL

Breakfast	Servings	Calories
		Subtotal
Snack		
		Subtotal
Lunch		
		Subtotal
Snack		
		Subtotal
Dinner		
		Subtotal
Snack		
		Subtotal

Total Calories From Food

FITNESS ACTIVITY JOURNAL

	Duration	Calories

Total Calories From Fitness

NOTES

FOOD JOURNAL

Breakfast	Servings	Calories
	Subtotal	

Snack		
	Subtotal	

Lunch		
	Subtotal	

Snack		
	Subtotal	

Dinner		
	Subtotal	

Snack		
	Subtotal	

Total Calories From Food [ ]

FITNESS ACTIVITY JOURNAL

	Duration	Calories

Total Calories From Fitness [ ]

NOTES

FOOD JOURNAL

Breakfast	Servings	Calories
	Subtotal	

Snack		
	Subtotal	

Lunch		
	Subtotal	

Snack		
	Subtotal	

Dinner		
	Subtotal	

Snack		
	Subtotal	

Total Calories From Food [   ]

FITNESS ACTIVITY JOURNAL

	Duration	Calories

Total Calories From Fitness [   ]

NOTES

FOOD JOURNAL

Breakfast		Servings	Calories	
			Subtotal	
Snack				
			Subtotal	
Lunch				
			Subtotal	
Snack				
			Subtotal	
Dinner				
			Subtotal	
Snack				
			Subtotal	
		Total Calories From Food		

FITNESS ACTIVITY JOURNAL

	Duration	Calories
Total Calories From Fitness		

NOTES

FOOD JOURNAL

Breakfast	Servings	Calories
	Subtotal	

Snack		
	Subtotal	

Lunch		
	Subtotal	

Snack		
	Subtotal	

Dinner		
	Subtotal	

Snack		
	Subtotal	

Total Calories From Food

FITNESS ACTIVITY JOURNAL

	Duration	Calories

Total Calories From Fitness

NOTES

FOOD JOURNAL

Breakfast	Servings	Calories
	Subtotal	

Snack		
	Subtotal	

Lunch		
	Subtotal	

Snack		
	Subtotal	

Dinner		
	Subtotal	

Snack		
	Subtotal	

Total Calories From Food

FITNESS ACTIVITY JOURNAL

	Duration	Calories

Total Calories From Fitness

NOTES

FOOD JOURNAL

Breakfast	Servings	Calories
	Subtotal	

Snack		
	Subtotal	

Lunch		
	Subtotal	

Snack		
	Subtotal	

Dinner		
	Subtotal	

Snack		
	Subtotal	

Total Calories From Food

FITNESS ACTIVITY JOURNAL

	Duration	Calories

Total Calories From Fitness

NOTES

FOOD JOURNAL

Breakfast	Servings	Calories
	Subtotal	

Snack		
	Subtotal	

Lunch		
	Subtotal	

Snack		
	Subtotal	

Dinner		
	Subtotal	

Snack		
	Subtotal	

Total Calories From Food

FITNESS ACTIVITY JOURNAL

	Duration	Calories

Total Calories From Fitness

NOTES

FOOD JOURNAL

Breakfast		Servings	Calories
		Subtotal	
Snack			
		Subtotal	
Lunch			
		Subtotal	
Snack			
		Subtotal	
Dinner			
		Subtotal	
Snack			
		Subtotal	
	Total Calories From Food		

FITNESS ACTIVITY JOURNAL

	Duration	Calories
Total Calories From Fitness		

NOTES

FOOD JOURNAL

Breakfast	Servings	Calories	
		Subtotal	

Snack			
		Subtotal	

Lunch			
		Subtotal	

Snack			
		Subtotal	

Dinner			
		Subtotal	

Snack			
		Subtotal	

Total Calories From Food

FITNESS ACTIVITY JOURNAL

	Duration	Calories

Total Calories From Fitness

NOTES

FOOD JOURNAL

Breakfast	Servings	Calories
	Subtotal	

Snack		
	Subtotal	

Lunch		
	Subtotal	

Snack		
	Subtotal	

Dinner		
	Subtotal	

Snack		
	Subtotal	

Total Calories From Food

FITNESS ACTIVITY JOURNAL

	Duration	Calories

Total Calories From Fitness

NOTES

FOOD JOURNAL

Breakfast	Servings	Calories
	Subtotal	

Snack		
	Subtotal	

Lunch		
	Subtotal	

Snack		
	Subtotal	

Dinner		
	Subtotal	

Snack		
	Subtotal	

Total Calories From Food [   ]

FITNESS ACTIVITY JOURNAL

	Duration	Calories

Total Calories From Fitness [   ]

NOTES

FOOD JOURNAL

Breakfast	Servings	Calories
	Subtotal	

Snack		
	Subtotal	

Lunch		
	Subtotal	

Snack		
	Subtotal	

Dinner		
	Subtotal	

Snack		
	Subtotal	

Total Calories From Food

FITNESS ACTIVITY JOURNAL

	Duration	Calories

Total Calories From Fitness

NOTES

FOOD JOURNAL

Breakfast	Servings	Calories
	Subtotal	

Snack		
	Subtotal	

Lunch		
	Subtotal	

Snack		
	Subtotal	

Dinner		
	Subtotal	

Snack		
	Subtotal	

Total Calories From Food

FITNESS ACTIVITY JOURNAL

	Duration	Calories

Total Calories From Fitness

NOTES

FOOD JOURNAL

Breakfast	Servings	Calories
	Subtotal	

Snack		
	Subtotal	

Lunch		
	Subtotal	

Snack		
	Subtotal	

Dinner		
	Subtotal	

Snack		
	Subtotal	

Total Calories From Food [   ]

FITNESS ACTIVITY JOURNAL

	Duration	Calories

Total Calories From Fitness [   ]

NOTES

FOOD JOURNAL

Breakfast	Servings	Calories
	Subtotal	

Snack		
	Subtotal	

Lunch		
	Subtotal	

Snack		
	Subtotal	

Dinner		
	Subtotal	

Snack		
	Subtotal	

	Total Calories From Food	

FITNESS ACTIVITY JOURNAL

	Duration	Calories
Total Calories From Fitness		

NOTES

FOOD JOURNAL

Breakfast	Servings	Calories
	Subtotal	

Snack		
	Subtotal	

Lunch		
	Subtotal	

Snack		
	Subtotal	

Dinner		
	Subtotal	

Snack		
	Subtotal	

Total Calories From Food _____

FITNESS ACTIVITY JOURNAL

	Duration	Calories

Total Calories From Fitness _____

NOTES

FOOD JOURNAL

Breakfast	Servings	Calories	
		Subtotal	

Snack			
		Subtotal	

Lunch			
		Subtotal	

Snack			
		Subtotal	

Dinner			
		Subtotal	

Snack			
		Subtotal	

		Total Calories From Food	

FITNESS ACTIVITY JOURNAL

	Duration	Calories
	Total Calories From Fitness	

NOTES

FOOD JOURNAL

Breakfast	Servings	Calories
	Subtotal	

Snack		
	Subtotal	

Lunch		
	Subtotal	

Snack		
	Subtotal	

Dinner		
	Subtotal	

Snack		
	Subtotal	

Total Calories From Food

FITNESS ACTIVITY JOURNAL

	Duration	Calories

Total Calories From Fitness

NOTES

FOOD JOURNAL

Breakfast	Servings	Calories	
		Subtotal	

Snack			
		Subtotal	

Lunch			
		Subtotal	

Snack			
		Subtotal	

Dinner			
		Subtotal	

Snack			
		Subtotal	

Total Calories From Food

FITNESS ACTIVITY JOURNAL

	Duration	Calories

Total Calories From Fitness

NOTES

FOOD JOURNAL

Breakfast	Servings	Calories
		Subtotal
Snack		
		Subtotal
Lunch		
		Subtotal
Snack		
		Subtotal
Dinner		
		Subtotal
Snack		
		Subtotal

Total Calories From Food

FITNESS ACTIVITY JOURNAL

	Duration	Calories

Total Calories From Fitness

NOTES

FOOD JOURNAL

Breakfast	Servings	Calories	
		Subtotal	

Snack			
		Subtotal	

Lunch			
		Subtotal	

Snack			
		Subtotal	

Dinner			
		Subtotal	

Snack			
		Subtotal	

Total Calories From Food

FITNESS ACTIVITY JOURNAL

	Duration	Calories

Total Calories From Fitness

NOTES

FOOD JOURNAL

Breakfast	Servings	Calories
	Subtotal	

Snack		
	Subtotal	

Lunch		
	Subtotal	

Snack		
	Subtotal	

Dinner		
	Subtotal	

Snack		
	Subtotal	

Total Calories From Food

FITNESS ACTIVITY JOURNAL

	Duration	Calories

Total Calories From Fitness

NOTES

FOOD JOURNAL

Breakfast	Servings	Calories
	Subtotal	

Snack		
	Subtotal	

Lunch		
	Subtotal	

Snack		
	Subtotal	

Dinner		
	Subtotal	

Snack		
	Subtotal	

Total Calories From Food

FITNESS ACTIVITY JOURNAL

	Duration	Calories

Total Calories From Fitness

NOTES

FOOD JOURNAL

Breakfast		Servings	Calories
		Subtotal	

Snack			
		Subtotal	

Lunch			
		Subtotal	

Snack			
		Subtotal	

Dinner			
		Subtotal	

Snack			
		Subtotal	

Total Calories From Food

FITNESS ACTIVITY JOURNAL

	Duration	Calories

Total Calories From Fitness

NOTES

FOOD JOURNAL

Breakfast	Servings	Calories
	Subtotal	

Snack		
	Subtotal	

Lunch		
	Subtotal	

Snack		
	Subtotal	

Dinner		
	Subtotal	

Snack		
	Subtotal	

Total Calories From Food

FITNESS ACTIVITY JOURNAL

	Duration	Calories

Total Calories From Fitness

NOTES

FOOD JOURNAL

Breakfast	Servings	Calories
		Subtotal

Snack		
		Subtotal

Lunch		
		Subtotal

Snack		
		Subtotal

Dinner		
		Subtotal

Snack		
		Subtotal

Total Calories From Food [   ]

FITNESS ACTIVITY JOURNAL

	Duration	Calories

Total Calories From Fitness [   ]

NOTES

FOOD JOURNAL

Breakfast	Servings	Calories
	Subtotal	

Snack		
	Subtotal	

Lunch		
	Subtotal	

Snack		
	Subtotal	

Dinner		
	Subtotal	

Snack		
	Subtotal	

Total Calories From Food

FITNESS ACTIVITY JOURNAL

	Duration	Calories

Total Calories From Fitness

NOTES

FOOD JOURNAL

Breakfast	Servings	Calories
	Subtotal	

Snack		
	Subtotal	

Lunch		
	Subtotal	

Snack		
	Subtotal	

Dinner		
	Subtotal	

Snack		
	Subtotal	

Total Calories From Food

FITNESS ACTIVITY JOURNAL

	Duration	Calories

Total Calories From Fitness

NOTES

Printed in Great Britain
by Amazon

53912466R00056